First Medicinal Alkaline Diets & Herbs

for Stubborn Sexually Transmitted Diseases (STDs) with Dr. Sebi Attributes

Liftmeh Genyus

Copyright © 2020

Table of Contents

Introduction

Sexually transmitted diseases (STDs) are sometimes referred to as sexually transmitted infections (STI). STDs are diseases that can be transmitted through sexual intercourse. Sexually transmitted diseases contraction depends on the immunity system of the body. In other words, the lower the immunity of the body, the greater the risk of contracting sexually transmitted diseases.

The number of times you involve in unprotected sexual intercourse does not determine whether and how you contract these diseases as you may contract it the first time you involve in sex.

Furthermore, knowing who your partner is or are does not determine whether you will contract these diseases or not as your partner (s) might be infected without you knowing it. Hence, the handsomeness or prettiness of your partner does not indicate whether they have one or more sexually transmitted diseases.

Many individuals get infected with two or more types of sexually transmitted diseases at a time and can also obtain it more than once.

Sexually transmitted diseases cause a significant number of deaths and illnesses among young individuals, adults, and newborn babies.

Most individuals that have contracted STDs do not show any symptoms most especially in women. Asymptomatic people will not know they have STDs and therefore, remain with it for a long period without management. As a result, unknown infected individuals continue to infect the uninfected ones.

It is reported by the World Health Organization (WHO) that annually nearly 500 million new cases of syphilis, gonorrhea, chlamydia, and Trichomoniasis arise in men and women of ages 15 and 49 years, and the global incidence continues to increase.

The major groups of individuals that are affected by sexually transmitted diseases are adolescents. This is because adolescents are often at higher risk of acquiring it. Also, they cannot intellectualize actions and their subsequent consequences or aftermath effects.

Sexually transmitted diseases are more prevalent among women of adolescent age than men because females are also more susceptible to it. Also, women experience increased anatomical and physiological exposure to infection due to increased cervical issues.

The mode of transmission of the sexually transmitted disease is through the following: anal to anal sex, oral to anal sex, vaginal sex, and oral to oral sex; although, there are other means by which these diseases can be transmitted.

The different types of sexually transmitted diseases are HIV, genital herpes, chlamydia, gonorrhea, syphilis, Human Papillomavirus, pelvic inflammatory disease…and many others.

Many individuals have suffered for several years as a result of STDs without a cure because some types of these diseases are not curable conventionally.

As a result, some certain numbers of therapeutic alkaline herbs and diets that are capable of fighting herpes, HIV, and other STDs are identified. Therefore, in this book, the types, causes, symptoms, natural treatments, and diets that are effective for fighting these diseases will be discussed.

Enjoy reading this book and I want you to be rest assured that if you strictly follow the alkaline herbs and the processes involved in curing each disease you will obtain positive results.

Chapter 1

Sexually transmitted diseases (STDs) are occasionally referred to as sexually transmitted infections (STI). STDs are diseases that can be transmitted through sexual intercourse.

The number of times you involve in unprotected sexual intercourse does not determine whether and how you contract these diseases as you may contract it the first time you involve in sex.

Furthermore, knowing who your partner is or are does not determine whether you will contract these diseases or not as your partner (s) might be infected without you knowing it. Hence, the handsomeness or prettiness of your partner does not indicate whether they have one or more sexually transmitted diseases.

Many individuals get infected with two or more types of sexually transmitted diseases at a time and can also obtain it more than once.

Sexually transmitted diseases cause a significant number of deaths and illnesses among young individuals, adults, and newborn babies.

Most individuals that have contracted STDs do not show any symptoms most especially in women. Asymptomatic people will not know they have STDs and therefore, remain with it for a long period without management. As a result, unknown infected individuals continue to infect the uninfected ones.

It is reported by the World Health Organization (WHO) that annually nearly 500 million new cases of syphilis, gonorrhea, chlamydia, and Trichomoniasis arise in men and women of ages 15 and 49 years, and the global incidence continues to increase.

The major groups of individuals that are affected by sexually transmitted diseases are adolescents. This is because adolescents are often at higher risk of acquiring it. Also, they cannot intellectualize actions and their subsequent consequences or aftermath effects.

Sexually transmitted diseases are more prevalent among women of adolescent age than men because females are also more susceptible to it. Also, women experience increased anatomical and physiological exposure to infection due to increased cervical issues.

Types of Sexually Transmitted Diseases (STDs)

There are different types of sexually transmitted diseases. The most common types are:

- Human Immunodeficiency Virus (HIV).
- Genital herpes.
- Gonorrhea.
- Syphilis.
- Chlamydia.
- Pelvic inflammatory disease (PID).
- Hepatitis B and C.
- Trichomoniasis.
- Human papillomavirus (HPV).
- Pubic lice.

Let us look at each of these diseases in detail before we consider the treatments required.

Human Immunodeficiency Virus (HIV)

Human Immunodeficiency Virus is a sexually transmitted disease. It affects the immune system of the body. In other words, it attacks the cells that assist the human body to fight infections. When this happens, the individual that is infected becomes exposed to different types of diseases.

Mostly, this disease is contracted via a connection with body fluids with an infected. This fluid can be gotten via unprotected sexual intercourse or the use of sharp objects that are already infected with the virus.

Phases of Human Immunodeficiency Virus

The phases of the Human Immunodeficiency Virus are:

- Acute phase.
- Chronic phase.
- Acquired Immunodeficiency Syndrome (AIDS) phase.

Acute phase: in this stage, the virus is already present in the blood without showing symptoms and some individuals may have symptoms that are similar to flu.

However, symptoms that resemble that of flu does not mean you are infected with this virus. This virus at this stage could be highly contagious. It could also cause some people to feel sick

Chronic phase: at this stage, there is a high possibility of not showing symptoms at all. It could also be termed as dormancy stage. The dormancy stage shows little activities and the production rate is reduced.

Most individuals live for about 10 years in this stage without any problem. Some do not even take medication and they remain healthy for long although, they continue to transfer this infection to others unknowingly. At this stage, infected individuals must engage in protected sex to stop the spread of the virus.

More so, the dormancy stage shows a drastic increase in the amount of the virus in the body. This is why testing and treatment are important at this stage to prevent it from entering the final stage.

Acquired Immunodeficiency Syndrome (AIDS) Phase

The second stage of this virus advances to this stage known as AIDS. At this stage, the immune system is totally affected and this provides room for other foreign bodies (infectious diseases) to come in.

Here, the amount of virus is at its peak and the CD4 (white blood cells that help your body fight diseases) count reduces drastically which could be a result of other infections that the body has contracted.

Many infected individuals at this stage survive for many years with treatment but some die within two to three years without any form of management.

How it is spread and causes

HIV could be spread through the following:

- Having unprotected sexual intercourse.
- Breastfeeding, delivery of baby, and pregnancy.
- Using a needle that is previously used by an infected person.
- Blood transfusion.

Symptoms of HIV

The following are the symptoms of HIV:

- Chills.

- Oral yeast infection.

- Frequent fever.

- Chronic diarrhea.

- Swollen lymph glands.

- Persistent white spots on your tongue or in your mouth.

- Persistent, unexplained fatigue.

- Weakness.

- Night sweats.

- Weight loss.

- Skin rashes.

- Pneumonia.

- Swollen lymph nodes…and more.

HIV Infection Related Diseases

These are diseases that find their way into the body as a result of the immune system being compromised. Examples of these diseases are:

Candidiasis: This mostly affects the vagina in women that are affected by HIV but the diagnosis of Candidiasis in an individual does not mean the individual is HIV positive. Candidiasis acts as an opportunist infection when an individual is HIV infected. Also, it shows signs of thick white coating in the mouth, tongue, and esophagus.

Pneumocystis pneumonia: this infection also finds its way into the body of an HIV infected individual as an opportunistic infection. Pneumonia is a fungal infection. Note that you might have pneumonia without having HIV.

Tuberculosis: This is also an opportunist infection associated with HIV infection. Individuals infected with HIV require constant management in order to prevent the invasion of this infection into the body as it causes death especially when the infection is at the third stage (AIDS stage).

Cryptococcal meningitis: this occurs when the membranes and fluids surrounding the spinal cord and brain is swollen. This infection also acts as an opportunistic infection in a HIV infected individual.

Chapter 2

Genital Herpes

Genital herpes is a sexually transmitted disease (STD) that is caused by the herpes simplex virus. This herpes simplex virus is of two types: HSV-1 and HSV-2. HSV-2 is the major cause of genital herpes that is transmitted via different types of sex such as oral, anal, and vaginal sex.

This disease is most prevalent among women between ages 14-49. This shows that one woman among 5-6 women is infected with this virus. This is because women's bodies are very vulnerable to this virus.

Most individuals infected with genital herpes do not show symptoms, hence, the ability to transmit it unknowingly is at its increase.

This virus is spread through the following means:

- Contact with the vaginal.
- Child delivery.
- Breastfeeding of a child through the child touching the sores in the body.

- Vaginal, oral, or anal sexual intercourse. Genital herpes virus is commonly transmitted through contact with open sores.

Symptoms of Genital Herpes

The majority of people that have genital herpes are asymptomatic, hence, the ability to identify that they have is a problem.

Also, some people do show some mild to moderate symptoms without acknowledging the fact that they have genital herpes. Hence, they refuse to go any test or diagnosis. Therefore, some symptoms that could make you take a step of going for testing include:

- Ulcers in the genital region.
- Scabs.
- Pain in the genitals.
- Itching in the genital region.
- Red bumps.
- Genital sores.
- White blisters…and more.

Problems Associated with Genital Herpes

Some diseases are related to genital herpes. These diseases attack the body with the influence of genital herpes infection. Examples of genital herpes related complications are:

Bladder abnormalities: this could show a sign of inflammation in the bladder. This inflammation could close up the urethra thereby hindering the easy passage of urine. Sores in the genital region could subsequently result in the inflammation of the tubes that transfer urine from the bladder to the urethra.

Inflammation of the rectum: this usually occurs among men who are gay. Genital herpes can result in swelling of the lining of the rectal organ, especially among men that practice sexual intercourse with the same sex.

Additional Sexually transmitted diseases: genital herpes improves your risk of spreading or contracting additional sexually transmitted diseases.

Neonatal diseases: mothers who have genital herpes easily spread this disease to their babies especially during birth hence; the ability of the child to contract brain problems is at the increase. Some babies who are born blind or become blind at a particular age, contract this from their mothers most times.

Meningitis: some individuals that suffer from genital herpes or any other types of herpes simplex virus do experience inflammation of the membranes and cerebrospinal fluid surrounding the brain and spinal cord.

Gonorrhea

This infection usually affects the urethra, cervix, rectum, penis, anus, and vaginal. It is caused by bacteria gonorrhea. It is transmitted through sexual intercourse and it affects only humans.

Gonorrhea bacteria are found in the mucus of the penis, vaginal, throat, and rectum. Individuals who engage in sexual activities are capable of contracting this disease.

This disease is most prevalent among men and women of ages 15-30 who often engage in unprotected sexual intercourse. Again, individuals in this age have multiple sexes with multiple partners that do not show any symptoms. Gonorrhea is spread from women to men in about 20-25% but it is easily spread from men to women during sexual contact.

Furthermore, children contract this disease during birth from their mother. This is as a result of the baby passing through the vaginal tract that is infected. Children can also acquire this disease during molestation, especially when the male is infected.

In most cases, when women who are infected with this disease refuse to treat it, it may migrate through the endometrium to the oviduct thereby resulting in pelvic inflammatory disease (PID). Also, men who refuse to treat it experience the disease traveling through the urethra causing urethritis and epididymitis.

Transmission of Gonorrhea
The bacterial is found in the mucus of the vaginal and penis. It is transmitted via unprotected sexual intercourse and could also be spread through sex toys that are previously used by an infected person.

The bacteria can be transmitted from mother to child during child delivery.

Conditions that Makes you be at Risk of Having Gonorrhea

The conditions that can make you easily contract this bacterial infection include the following:

- When you have other untreated sexually transmitted diseases.
- When you have a new sex companion.
- When you have more than one sex companion.
- When you have a sex companion that has another sex companion.

Symptoms of Gonorrhea

- Pain during urination.
- Discharge from the vagina with an unpleasant smell.
- Abdominal or pelvic pain.
- Vaginal bleeding between periods, such as after vaginal intercourse.
- Fever.

- Irregular menstruation.

- Pain in the pelvis.

- Discharge of pus from the tip of the penis.

- Swelling of the testicle.

- The urgency in urinating.

- Pain in the lower abdomen.

- Pain in the testicle.

Chapter 3

Syphilis

Syphilis is caused by bacterium *Treponema pallidum*. Syphilis is known as a sexually transmitted disease that affects every man or woman who is sexually active. This infection is curable but the inability to undergo treatment will result in severe health problems.

This disease can be spread via close skin connection with an infected individual, through unprotected vaginal, anal, and oral sex with an infected person.

Also, this infection can be transmitted from mother to child during pregnancy and birth. Hence, pregnant women must undergo diagnosis to ensure they treat this infection properly to prevent spreading it to their children.

Stages of Syphilis

There are about four stages of syphilis. These stages are discussed below:

Stage 1 (primary stage): this stage is unset of syphilis. It shows a painless sore at the region of penetration of the bacteria. Most times, this lasts for about 3-4 weeks and at this stage, an infected individual can easily transmit it unknowingly because he/she is unaware.

The sore is mostly in the area surrounding the penis among men but women experience the sore at the innermost part of the vagina. This sore does not show any sign of pain, hence, you might not know you have syphilis.

In most cases, the lymph nodes that surround the sores may be inflamed. However, this sore can disappear without treatment but this does not mean the infection has disappeared. In this case, the individual can spread it to others.

Stage 2 (secondary): this shows some advances in symptoms other than sores. There is a characteristic rash that manifests after the manifestation of the sores. The rashes most times, migrate all over the body. The spread of this rash over the body shows symptoms such as sore throat, weight loss, inflammation of the lymph nodes, fever, weakness, patch hair loss, neck stiffness, headaches, paralysis, irritability…and more. Therefore, you have to undergo treatment when you discover all these symptoms as delay might be dangerous.

Stage 3 (latent): at this stage, the infected individuals might not have any symptoms. The rash, sores, and other signs are no longer visible because the symptoms are capable of going away without treatment even when the infection is still much active in the body. It is the only diagnosis that can identify that you have syphilis at this stage.

Stage 4 (tertiary): the tertiary stage is the most destructive stage of this disease. An infected individual that refuses to treat it might experience problems of cardiovascular syphilis, brain damage, eye problem, bone abnormalities...and more.

Risk Condition of Syphilis

The following are the people who are at risk of having syphilis:

- Those who have more than one sex partner.

- Men who have sex with men.

- Sex workers.

- When you have other sexually transmitted diseases.

- Pregnant women sexual partners that have other sex partners.

- Women who have sex with women.

Symptoms of Syphilis

The symptoms of syphilis include:

- Presence of a single sore that usually painless.

- Swollen lymph nodes

- Presence of flat, red skin rash on the soles of your feet, palms, or it may cover your entire body.

- Hair loss

- Pain in the joints or flu-like illness.

- Vision problems.

- Problems in the muscle.

- Nerve damage.

- Brain damage, dementia, and mental health problems.

- Heart disease.

- Movement syndromes.

- Seizures.

- Tumors on the skin.

Chlamydia

Chlamydia is a sexually transmitted disease that is caused by *Chlamydia trachomatis*. This is one of the most prevalent sexually transmitted disease in the United Kingdom and the United States.

This disease is prevalent among younger adults. It is spread from mother to children (congenital transmission) through an infected birth canal. It is spread from an infected person to an uninfected person via anal, oral, and vaginal sexual contact.

Chlamydia can cause problems related to childbirth ectopic pregnancy and can cause other diseases that are sexually transmitted. This disease can prevent women from getting pregnant because it causes damage to women's reproductive organs.

Most individuals who have this disease have no symptoms however, the symptoms show up as the bacteria progresses in the body.

Risk Condition of Chlamydia

The following are the factors that can make you be at risk of having chlamydia:

- When you have HIV.
- When you have a partner that is infected with chlamydia.
- When you have sex with men.
- When you have multiple sex partners.
- When you involve in unprotected sex with infected partners…and more.

Symptoms of Chlamydia

The following are the symptoms associated with Chlamydia:

- Vaginal discharge.
- Bleeding.
- Discharge from the penis.
- Burning sensation when urinating.

- Abnormal vaginal discharge.

- Burning sensation during urination.

- Pain in the rectum.

- Pain and inflammation in one or both testicles.

Pelvic Inflammatory Disease (PID)

This is a sexually transmitted disease that is caused by bacteria. This usually affects the female's ovaries, cervix, oviduct (fallopian tube), uterus, and vagina. This is one of the major reasons that prevent a woman from getting pregnant.

It is reported that more than one million women are infected with this disease in the United States and this has resulted in infertility in more than a hundred thousand women.

The pelvic inflammatory disease has resulted in several tubal pregnancies (pregnancy in the fallopian tube). This is a severe case that has caused premature death among women.

A woman can contract this disease if a bacterium migrates up from her vagina or cervix and into her reproductive organs.

Different types of bacteria cause this disease. Majorly, it is caused by infection from two common sexually transmitted diseases such as chlamydia and gonorrhea.

The risk factor and symptoms of pelvic inflammatory disease are similar to the symptoms of chlamydia and gonorrhea.

Hepatitis B and C

Hepatitis is the term used to describe liver inflammation that is caused by a virus. There are different types of Hepatitis but in this book, I am going to discuss the B and C virus hepatitis which could be spread via sexual contact.

Hepatitis B and C affect millions of people resulting in liver cirrhosis and cancer. Hepatitis is transmitted from an infected person to an uninfected person through contact with the blood or other body fluids, including semen and vaginal fluid of an infected person. It can also be contracted through kissing or sharing needles.

The hepatitis C virus is spread through direct contact with infected blood. More so, individuals with HIV mostly suffer from Hepatitis. It advances faster and causes more liver problems among people with HIV than among people without HIV.

This virus could be spread from one person to another via sexual intercourse, sharing needles or sharp objects. It could also be spread from infected mothers to children especially during pregnancy and birth.

Symptoms of Hepatitis

The following are the possible symptoms of hepatitis:

- Fatigue.
- Dark urine.
- Stomach pain.
- Pain in the joint.
- Fever.
- Jaundice.
- Vomiting.

- Diarrhea.

- Pale stool.

- Poor appetite.

Trichomoniasis

Trichomoniasis is a sexually transmitted disease that is caused by *Trichomonas vaginalis*. This infection usually affects females that are of sexual age than males.

It is reported that about 3.75 million individuals are infected with *Trichomonas vaginalis* in the United States. Also, women who are older contract this infection than younger women.

This infection causes foul smell in the vaginal discharge among women while men do not show any symptoms as the infection is asymptomatic in most men.

Trichomoniasis can intensify the risk of contracting or spreading other sexually transmitted diseases. This is the reason pregnant women must ensure they are free from this infection and other sexually transmitted diseases as it could be transmitted from mother to babies either during pregnancy or delivery.

Trichomoniasis could be spread through the following: unprotected vaginal sex, unprotected oral sex, and unprotected anal sex.

Symptoms of Trichomoniasis

The following are the symptoms of Trichomoniasis:

- Itching of the vaginal.

- Burning in the vaginal.

- Redness of the vaginal.

- Pain during urination.

- Heavy vaginal discharge with different colors such as green, white, yellow.

- Unpleasant vaginal discharge odor…and more.

Chapter 4

Sexually Transmitted Diseases (STDs) and Prevention

Sexually transmitted diseases could be very dangerous if left without treatment. Prevention is very cheap and better than a cure. This is why I am going to discuss more on the prevention of STDs.

Sexually transmitted diseases can be prevented through the following ways:

- Screen blood before transfusion.
- Encourage the use of condoms.
- Maintain a single-sex partner.
- Abstain from unprotected sex.
- Engage in the test before sex.
- Reduce the number of sex partners.
- Vaccination.
- Abstain from sex.

Screen blood before transfusion: sexually transmitted diseases such as HIV could be easily contracted or transmitted when an individual receives blood from an infected person. This is the reason it is important to screen blood before transfusion; although, transfusion of blood is not a route of transmitting sexually transmitted diseases the virus is in unscreened blood.

Encourage the use of condoms: the use of latex condoms is very important in preventing sexually transmitted diseases although, the use of condoms is not effective in preventing STDs 100% at least you will be on a safe side. However, you use condoms whenever you are having anal, oral, and vaginal sex.

Maintain a single-sex partner: to maintain a single-sex partner to prevent STDs, you must agree with your partner that both of you will only engage in sexual intercourse together without multiple sex partners. This is one of the most effective and reliable ways of preventing sexually transmitted diseases. However, the two of you must first go for testing to ensure you are both free from STDs.

Abstain from unprotected sex: unprotected sexual intercourse is one of the ways that makes you open to contracting sexually transmitted diseases. Hence, if you must engage in multiple sexes, ensure you use any mode of protection at least to be safe from contracting STDs.

Engage in a test before sex: ensure you engage in testing before having sex with your partner(s) because this will prevent you from contracting from others and spreading STDs to others. Tests can also help you to know your status and how to manage your sexual life.

Decrease the number of sex partners: decreasing the number of sex partners can help you drastically reduce the risk associated with having STDs.

Vaccination: vaccination is also one of the important, efficient, and safe ways of preventing some types of sexually transmitted diseases such as human papillomavirus and hepatitis B. although, these vaccines are only recommended for children between 9-26 years. Those who have not been vaccinated when they were younger can also do the same.

Abstain from sex: abstinence as far as I am concern is the major way of preventing sexually transmitted diseases. You can abstain from sex when you are not married and ensure you get tested with your partner before you begin the sexual relationships.

Diagnosis of Sexually Transmitted Diseases (STDs)

Diagnosis involves the examination of the body to detect if an individual has contracted any of the sexually transmitted diseases. The diagnoses of sexually transmitted diseases are discussed below:

Syphilis: this involves examining pelvic and medical history. Again, the following test can be conducted: Venereal Disease Research Laboratory blood test, Rapid Plasma Reagin blood test, Fluorescent Treponemal Antibody-Absorption antibody blood test, and T. pallidum hemagglutination assay, to confirm a positive finding on the blood.

Genital herpes: can be diagnosed through the following: Physical examination, herpes virus blood test, and culture.

HIV: HIV can be diagnosed through the following: Physical examination, Rapid HIV test completed on blood or saliva, ELISA (Enzyme-Linked Immunosorbent Assay) antibody blood test.

After the test has been conducted, the result will determine if there will be a need for further tests. Hence, if the sample tests positive for HIV, there will be a need to conduct an antibody blood test or an HIV nucleic acid test.

Gonorrhea: can be diagnosed through the following: Physical examination, pelvic examination, laboratory testing of cervical, vaginal secretion, and secretion of the penile region.

Pelvic inflammatory disease (PID): can be diagnosed through the following: Physical examination, laboratory tests of cervical or vaginal secretions, ultrasound imaging exam.

Chlamydia: chlamydia can be diagnosed through the following: Physical examination, pelvic examination analysis of cervical secretions or urine, to examine the presence of C. trachomatis.

Human Papilloma Virus (HPV): can be diagnosed through the following: Physical examination, Pap smear or colposcopy, and cervical biopsy…and many more.

Are Acidic Foods Good for STDs?

The answer to this question is the capital 'NO'. Acidic foods are capable of making the body vulnerable to the contraction of diseases because many diseases causing-organisms thrive well in an acidic environment. This is what makes the alkaline diet the most superior diet that is very effective for the prevention, reverse, and cure of diseases.

In lieu of this, sufferers of STDs who adopt an alkaline diet can raise their pH levels, which caused the HIV or Herpes cells to become inactive or latent.

Alkaline Diets and Sexually Transmitted Diseases (STDs)

Alkaline diets are diets that are free from acid. An alkaline body is capable of fighting against diseases like STDs and provides an environment that helps in preventing the invasion of disease-causing organisms.

Sustaining proper alkaline levels in the body is vital for overall good health as well as preventing all sexually transmitted diseases outbreaks.

In other words, disease-causing organisms cherish environments that are acidic because of the spread and multiply easily in such an environment.

The alkaline diet performs its functions by self-healing the body. Hence, for the body to heal itself it requires the right factors such as the right pH, adequate nutrients, exercise, and water.

The major factor that affects our pH is the foods we eat. Through consuming alkaline foods and reducing acidic foods, our bodies can start to prevent diseases, heal the body, and help protect from external acid factors like stress and radiation.

Ultimately, the pH of the body is very important in order to have healthy wellbeing. In order to retain a healthy pH in the body, the need to eat at least 70% alkaline foods is essential.

Alkaline foods include most cooked and raw vegetables, fruits, grains, herbs, nuts, and spices. Acidic foods include meat, dairy, sugar, processed foods, coffee, grains, and nuts. There is much-supporting research that shows that an alkaline diet can support health.

Chapter 5

The Alkaline Diet as Case in point

This alkaline diet has been a diet of interest for me and my family for the past seven years. I stumbled on the diet when I heard about a man called Doctor Sebi. Dr. Sebi was a herbal practitioner and a natural therapist who used alkaline herbs and diets to treat several diseases including HIV, Herpes, Cancer, Hepatitis, Syphilis, and all other STDS.

In the course of this write-up, I will shortly show you the examples of Dr. Sebi's alkaline diets and herbs (food lists).

The Recommended Alkaline Vegetable foods: Nopales, Nori, Zucchini, Lettuce except for iceberg, Wild Arugula, Watercress, Wakame, Red Onions, Arame, Avocado, Bell Pepper, Chayote, Cucumber, Cherry and Plum Tomato, Green Amaranth, Dandelion Greens, Dulse, Garbanzo Beans, Izote flower and leaf, Turnip

Greens, Squash, Okra, Tomatillo, Kale, Olives, Purslane Verdolaga, Mushrooms except for Shitake and Hijiki.

The Recommended Alkaline Fruits: Prunes, Figs, Prickly Pear, Peaches, Soft Jelly Coconuts, Pears, Plums, Soursops, Dates, Raisins, Currants, Orange, Limes, Papayas, Cantaloupe, Melons, Bananas, Cherries, Grapes, Apples, Mango and Berries.

The Recommended Alkaline Spices and Seasonings: Basil, Thyme, Pure Sea Salt, Powdered Granulated Seaweed, Achiote, Habanero, Savory, Cayenne, Sweet Basil, Onion Powder, Oregano, Sage, Tarragon, Cloves, Dill and Bay Leaf.

The Recommended Alkaline Grains: Quinoa, Fonio, Amaranth, Wild Rice, Tef, Spelt, Kamut, and Rye.

The Recommended Alkaline Sugar: Dried Date Sugar and 100% Pure Agave Syrup from cactus.

The Recommended Alkaline Herbs: Basil, Onion powder, Dill, Oregano, Cayenne, and Pure sea salt.

The Recommended Alkaline Herbal Tea: Tila, Red Raspberry, Chamomile, Elderberry, Ginger, Fennel, and Burdock.

The Benefits of Alkaline Diets

When acidic foods are reduced in your food, it builds an environment that makes it easy to fight against diseases and prevent the attack of disease-causing organisms in the body. Therefore, the benefits of alkaline diets are:

- Alkaline diets help in treating STDs perfectly.
- Alkaline diets help in the prevention and treatment of all types of cancer.
- Alkaline diets do not contain alcohol.
- Alkaline diets do not contain processed sugar.
- An alkaline diet boosts the immune system.
- Alkaline diets help in improving weight loss as a result of natural vegetables, fruits grains, and other organic foods.
- Alkaline diets have very low saturated fat for preventing and fighting heart-related diseases.
- Alkaline diets have completely no cholesterol.

- An alkaline diet reduces the risk of contracting diseases.

- The alkaline diet provides the body with the energy it required.

- Alkaline diets help brain function.

- The alkaline diet has very low fat which prevents heart diseases.

- Alkaline diet prevents and combats Diabetes.

- An alkaline diet prevents and treats stroke.

The Non-Alkaline Acidic Diets

The non-alkaline diets are the acidic diets and these diets must be shunned if the treatment of STDs is your priority. These diets are:

- Soy and soy products.

- Corn.

- Genetically Modified Organism fruits.

- Eggs.

- Processed foods.

- Canned foods and fruits.

- Wheat.

- Seedless fruits.

- Alcoholic beverages.

- Fish and seafood.

- The meat of all kinds.

- Foods fortified with vitamins and minerals

- Garlic.

- Genetically Modified Organism vegetables.

- Dairy foods.

- Poultry products.

- Colorants and flavors.

- Foods with yeast or another component such as baking powder.

- Fast foods.

- Sugar.

Chapter 6

Alkaline Herbs and Diets for Sexually Transmitted Diseases (STDs)

There are different types of herbs that are can treat different diseases but there are several alkaline herbs that are super capable and effective in treating all types of sexually transmitted diseases.

The alkaline herbs responsible for treating each disease will be described as follows:

Alkaline Herbs for HIV

There are different herbs that can help in fighting this virus. These herbs are:

- European mistletoe leaf.
- Echinacea.
- Dandelion root.
- Licorice.

Dandelion root

It is reported that dandelion obstructs the replication and multiplication of the Human Immunodeficiency Virus (HIV). Human Immunodeficiency Virus replication is responsible for the improvement of Acquired Immunodeficiency Syndrome in the body.

Licorice

Licorice performs its functions by acting as immunomodulation agents and antiviral agents. This plant has been used in different regions for the treatment of HIV for many years and clinical trials prove that it is very effective for suppressing the viral load of this virus in the body.

Echinacea: This plant is a very common herb that is used by the Native Americans to boosts the immune system of the body.

European mistletoe leaf: this plant is very effective against the inhibition of HIV toxicity in the human body.

How to prepare the herbs and dosage

You can prepare the above-recommended herbs in the following ways:

- Dry and preserve in a dry, clean, airtight container separately.
- Prepare each of the herbs into powder form.
- Collect half teaspoonful of each of the herbs and add four cups of alkaline water.
- Put on boiling kettle and allow it to boil for 5 minutes.
- Remove it from the heat source and leave it for a few minutes to get cool.
- Drain and drink.
- Take these herbs two times daily with a glass cup until your required result is achieved.

Alkaline Herbs for Genital Herpes

There are different herbs that can help in fighting this virus. These herbs are:

- Dandelion.
- Kale.

- Sarsil berry.

- Blue Vervain.

- Yellow dock.

- Burdock.

- Guaco.

- Concerns.

- Purslane.

- Sarsaparilla.

Guaco Plant: guaco plant contains an increased amount of iron that helps in strengthening the immune system and it is also loaded with potassium phosphate that makes it effective against genital herpes virus in the body.

Sarsaparilla: Sarsaparilla contains the highest iron component and it is used for treating genital herpes.

It is reported that sarsaparilla has mechanisms that help it to treat syphilis, herpes, rheumatic affections, passive general dropsy, and gonorrheal rheumatism.

The active ingredients present in this plant that makes it effective against herpes and many other STDs are triterpenes, sarsaparilloside, parillin, smitilbin, and phenolic components.

Sarsil Berry: Sarsil Berry is loaded with iron as it is a berry from the plant of Sarsaparilla. Dr. Sebi spoke comprehensively about this plant and pointed on its effectiveness for the cure of genital herpes simplex virus.

Conconsa: Conconsa is an African plant. The highest concentration of potassium phosphate is present in it. It also fights against the herpes virus.

Kale plant: Kale plant is loaded with iron and antioxidants. It is also loaded with abundant lysine. Lysine is an amino acid ratio that is essential in suppressing genital herpes virus. It helps in hindering the multiplication of herpes virus in the body of an infected individual.

How to prepare the herbs and dosage
You can prepare the above-listed herbs in the following ways:

- Dry and preserve in a dry, clean, airtight container separately.

- Prepare each of the herbs into powder form.

- Collect one teaspoonful of each of the plants and add four cups of alkaline water.

- Put on boiling kettle and allow it to boil for 5 minutes.

- Remove it from the heat source and leave it for a few minutes to get cool.

- Drain and drink.

- Take these herbs two times daily with a glass cup until your required result is achieved.

Alkaline Herbs for Trichomoniasis, Gonorrhea, and Syphilis

Examples of the herbs used for the treatment of *Trichomonas vaginalis* are:

Silybum marianum: this herb is employed for the treatment of STDs in the form of traditional medicine. The herb is rich in silymarin (a natural material that can destroy *T. vaginalis*), which makes the plant an ideal choice to fight against certain types of STDs.

Also, this component is used to increase the immunity of the body and therefore helps fight the parasite that causes infection.

Soma: soma is an effective herb for STDs especially Trichomoniasis due to its potent antibacterial properties. Leaves, tree bark, roots, and fruit of soma have high therapeutic importance, and its anti-inflammatory and antibacterial properties help in fighting several diseases such as gonorrhea and syphilis.

The active ingredient in this herb is saponin. Saponin consists of phytochemicals that help in killing all types of germs, boost the immune system, and re-energize the body.

Eucalyptus: eucalyptus has been suggested for the treatment of gonorrhea, with a very encouraging result. The oil of this herb reveals antimicrobial properties against different strains of bacteria. Ultimately, the antimicrobial effects of this plant are comparatively greater on gram-positive bacteria.

How to prepare the herbs and dosage

You can prepare the above-listed herbs in the following ways:

- Dry and preserve in a dry, clean, airtight container separately.
- Prepare each of the herbs into powder form.
- Collect one teaspoonful of each of the plants and add three cups of alkaline water.
- Put on boiling kettle and allow it to boil for 3-4 minutes.
- Remove it from the heat source and leave it for a few minutes to get cool.
- Drain and drink.
- Take these herbs two times daily with a glass cup until your required result is achieved.

Chapter 7

Alkaline Diets for other Sexually Transmitted Diseases

There are certain numbers of herbs that are effective for the treatment of other sexually transmitted diseases. These herbs are:

- Bitter Melon Edible Part (without Seed).

- Nauclea (Bark & Stem).

- Aleo vera (Leaf).

- Akuamma (seed).

- Spring Onion.

- Sword lily or Gladiolus Bulb.

- Coconut water/Lime juice.

- Euphorbia Herbs.

How to Prepare the Herbs

Bitter Melon

- Rinse the fruit and use a knife to remove the hard coat of the fruit.

- Divide the edible white region into four equal parts to remove all the embedded seeds.
- Thinly cube it and collect 2 cups of bitter Melon and keep it aside.

Nauclea (Bark or Stem)

- Collect an uninfected fresh Nauclea stem.
- Rinse the plant, chop and grind them.
- Pour all the pounded stems into a close container.
- Cover the container tightly and keep it on a platform like a kitchen shelf, cabinet, or cupboard. This will prevent moisture on the herbs.
- Allow it to infuse for three days drinking it.

Aloe vera: Rinse Aloe vera with clean water, thinly dice it, and take one cupful and keep it aside.

Akuamma Seed:

- Take away the coat of the seeds.
- Grind the seed and dry them with the use of sunlight or use hot air oven to dry them. However,

if the seeds are dried, directly grind them to powder after you have removed them from their coats.

Spring Onion:

- Thoroughly rinse the whole part of the Spring Onion.
- Ensure the leaf and bulb region are thoroughly rinsed.
- Dice the Spring Onion and quantify half cup and keep it at the side.

Gladiolus Bulb:

- Remove the leaves that cover the bulb.
- Rinse it with clean water.
- Dice and measure a quarter cup of it.

Dosages for Minor Condition

- Collect 5 tablespoons from the extract and drink before breakfast.

Dosages for Chronic Condition

- Collect 7 tablespoons from the extract and drink before a meal in the morning only.
- Drink it for 14days consecutively without any intermittent break, if you have used the extract to a ¼ of the container; add more of Coconut water to the half of the container.

Dosages for Prevention

- You can use the remaining medicine to prevent recurrence from taking about 3-4 tablespoons of the medicinal extract before breakfast or after dinner.

Preparation of Powdered Medicine

- Get all the ingredients mentioned above.
- Dry and preserve in a dry, clean, airtight container separately.
- Prepare each of the herbs into powder form.
- Collect one teaspoonful of each of the plants and add four cups of alkaline water.
- Put on boiling kettle and allow it to boil for 5 minutes.

- Remove it from the heat source and leave it for a few minutes to get cool.

- Drain and drink.

- Take these herbs two times daily with a glass cup until your required result is achieved.

Tips and Facts about Alkaline Herbs for STDs

- Eat foods that are listed in the food lists that are listed above.

- Do not eat foods that are non-alkaline diets.

- Desist from taking alcohol.

- You can engage in fasting if you can because it helps in removing excess deposits of fat in the body.

- Stick to the above listed alkaline diets.

- Continue with the intake of the alkaline fruits until your desired result is achieved.

References

Healthychildren.org. American Academy of pediatrics 2015.

Mohammedreza Nazer, Saber Abbaszadeh, Mona Moghadasi. The Most Important Herbs Used in the Treatment of Sexually Transmitted Infections in Traditional Medicine. Sudan Journal of Medical Sciences.

Dashtdar, M., Dashtdar, M. R., Dashtdar, B., et al. (2013). In-vitro, anti-bacterial activities of aqueous extracts of Acacia catechu (LF) Willd, Castanea sativa, Ephedra sinica Stapf, and shilajita mumiyo against Gram-positive and Gram-negative bacteria. Journal of Pharmacopuncture, vol. 16, no. 2: pp. 15–22.

Sheldon R. Morris (2019). Gonorrhea MSD Manual professional version.

Centers for Disease Control and Prevention. (2014). Sexually transmitted diseases in women and infants.

Kazhila C. Chinsembu. Sexually Transmitted Infections in Adolescents. The Open Infectious Diseases Journal, 2009, 3, 107-117.

Maroyi, A. (2017). Exotic plants in the indigenous pharmacopeia of south-central Zimbabwe: traditional knowledge of herbal medicines. Research Journal of Botany, vol. 12, no. 2, pp. 46–52.

Trivedi, J., et al. (2019). "Plant-Derived Molecules in Managing HIV Infection," in New Look to Phytomedicine, pp. 273–298. Cambridge, MA: Academic Press.

DRSEBICELLFOOD.COM